Reversing Peripheral Neuropathy

By Dr. Cory Aplin, D.C.

First Edition

ISBN: 978-1519363558

Printed in the United States of America

Table of Contents

Editor's Note

This book, *Reversing Peripheral Neuropathy,* is two books in one, or rather it is one book printed twice.

The first (approx.) half is the book printed with normal lay-out conventions which makes it the easiest way for many people to read the book.

Peripheral Neuropathy, as you will learn, afflicts a wide range of people. A good many have their best eyesight behind them. To address this we have changed the lay-out and have adopted larger print and formatting rules that are the latest in easy to read type.

The book has then been reprinted, exactly, again.

The easy to read version begins on page 71.

Introduction

"Peripheral nerves have the ability to regenerate axons, as long as the nerve cell itself has not died, which may lead to functional recovery over time"

-National Institute of Neurologic Disorders and Stroke on the topic of Peripheral Neuropathy

I start the introduction to this book with the above quote because nearly every patient who comes into my office has heard from at least one doctor (and usually multiple doctors) that:

1) There is nothing that can be done for Peripheral Neuropathy other than medication to manage symptoms.

2) Their condition will only get worse.

3) Nerves can't regenerate.

They come for their initial examination with a skeptical mind but out of desperation to find some relief (ANY relief) from the pain, numbness, tingling and/or burning in their feet. For most, nothing else they have tried has seemed to be able to help.

So I start with this quote to inspire hope! One of the most prominent authorities on neurologic disorders, a division of the National Institute of Health is saying, "Yes, peripheral nerves can regenerate", and "Yes, nerves damaged due to peripheral neuropathy can return to normal function".

It's an exciting job I have to be able to restore hope to those who feel hopeless. To deliver treatment options to those who thought there were none.

In this book, *Reversing Peripheral Neuropathy*, you will learn about the many causes of peripheral neuropathy, why traditional approaches to treatment have failed, and what can be done to take back control of your condition and your life.

Chapter 1: What is Peripheral Neuropathy?

Peripheral Neuropathy is a condition in which a person experiences pain, numbness, tingling, burning and/or weakness, usually in the hands and feet, though it may occur in other parts of the body.

The word itself betrays the general and somewhat mysterious nature of the disease. "Neuro", meaning related to nerves and "-pathy", pertaining to a disease or ailment. In medical circles, one can see that a lot of different conditions could be attributed to "something wrong with the nerves."

Regardless of the vague definition, peripheral neuropathy (also sometimes referred to as polyneuropathy) is typically diagnosed when a person has pain or numbness where there is no direct or observable cause for it.

This can occur as a result of nerve damage in the peripheral nervous system, which essentially encompasses all parts of the nervous system outside of the brain and spinal cord (i.e. spinal nerves).

These nerves are responsible for communicating information from the body back through the spinal cord and eventually to the brain.

As the nerves become more and more damaged, the normal signals become muted (numbness, weakness), or altered (pain, tingling, burning). These types of "nerve symptoms" are signs that the nerves are beginning to die.

There are 3 main types of nerves that can be affected to varying degrees:

Autonomic nerves: These regulate heart rate, sweating, blood pressure and other automatic functions of the body.

Motor nerves: These control the body muscles and are usually under conscious control.

Sensory nerves: These transmit sensations (such as pain, touch, heat and cold) from other body parts to the brain.

Some peripheral neuropathy sufferers will exhibit symptoms related to only one of these nerve types, while others will have symptoms related to two nerve types, and still others will show signs and symptoms of damage to all 3 nerve types.

Read on to find more on some of the common causes of this condition.

Chapter 2: Diagnosing Peripheral Neuropathy

There are over 100 causes and dozens of symptoms that can be associated with peripheral neuropathy, so it is important that the clinician be familiar with all of them in order to make the appropriate clinical correlation.

Many diabetic patients or those in the early stages of peripheral neuropathy are often asymptomatic (no symptoms). However, properly trained healthcare professionals can still identify slight tell-tale signs of the condition.

Specialized clinical tests can help determine what the general health condition of the patient is.

It may reveal the underlying cause of your peripheral neuropathy which will aid the doctor in developing an appropriate treatment plan and what the expected outcomes will be after treatment.

Physicians look out for the following Diabetic Neuropathy symptoms:

- Reduced ankle reflexes
- Painless foot injuries
- Infections
- Gangrene

Diagnosing peripheral neuropathy usually starts with a symptoms survey. This will give the clinician a detailed account of what you are experiencing and how it has changed or progressed over time.

The next step in diagnosing peripheral neuropathy is to perform a detailed neurological exam. Although this exam is comprehensive, it is fairly straightforward and does not necessarily require expensive equipment or scans.

In my office we use tried and true methods of determining to what degree you can still feel the affected limbs. We test your ability to feel vibration, temperature, tactile and other sensory perceptions.

These methods are all simple yet very effective in determining which nerves have been affected by your peripheral neuropathy and to what degree. Many of our patients are shocked to see first-hand how far along their peripheral neuropathy has progressed!

Using a standard scoring system we can then calculate how much function you have lost in your peripheral nerves. This gives us an objective measure to easily track your progress throughout the treatment.

We then use a highly specialized foot scanner to take a 3-D image of your foot. This gives us an up close view to evaluate for ulcers or other changes to the structure of the feet.

It measures pressure from side to side so we can evaluate specific pressure points, which may be relieved with specialized orthotic devices. Lastly, it measures the heat signature across the foot. An area of increased heat is a tell-tale sign of increased inflammation which helps us to determine a starting point for delivering treatment.

Other Diagnostic Methods

In Neurology offices, sometimes electro-diagnostic tools are used to assess peripheral neuropathies.

The first is called an Electromyogram, or EMG for short. This test measures the electrical activity of the muscles.

The second is called Nerve Conduction Velocity Study, or NCV for short. This test measures how fast a nerve can send an electric signal.

These two tests together are useful in determining the overall health of the muscles and nerves. They can show which nerves are affected by peripheral neuropathy and to what extent they have been affected.

By using electrodiagnostics, the doctor can determine an expected prognosis for the patient. As long as there is still some nerve function, it tells us that the nerve is not completely dead, meaning that the prognosis for recovery is good. If there is no nerve function, meaning that the lesion is definitive, recovery will be limited.

In either case, early intervention is key in maximizing results with treatment.

Chapter 3: What Causes Peripheral Neuropathy?

Peripheral neuropathy is relatively common in people over the age of 55. Approximately 4% to 6% of the people in this age group showed signs and symptoms of the disorder. Those with metabolic syndromes like diabetes are at a significantly greater risk with estimates that over 50% of diabetics suffer from peripheral neuropathy to some degree.

Over 100 different types of peripheral neuropathy have been identified and it is caused by many different underlying conditions.

In most cases, the disease damages nerves in the peripheral nervous system, usually in the hands and feet, but spares the brain and spinal cord.

Causes of peripheral neuropathy can be divided into 3 main categories: Disease type,

Exposure type and Traumatic type, which we will discuss in this chapter.

It is important to note that although these 3 categories exist, many cases of peripheral neuropathy are considered "idiopathic", meaning that there is no known cause.

The symptoms and effects of idiopathic peripheral neuropathy are the same as those found in other neuropathy sufferers, and treatments are equally effective across the groups.

Regardless of which category your peripheral neuropathy falls into, one of the root causes is damage to the small blood vessels that supply the nerves.

This starves the nerve of essential oxygen and nutrients which in turn results in nerve damage and the eventual dying off of the nerve.

Think of it as if the peripheral nerves in your hands or feet were like the roots of a tree and your blood supply is the tree's water source. What would happen if you stopped watering the roots of a tree?

It would start to die! And that is exactly what happens to your nerves when they are starved of their blood supply. The symptoms associated with peripheral neuropathy are a result of this withering of the nerves. This is an important point to remember for later in the book when I discuss different treatment options.

Besides being starved of oxygen, systemic diseases may affect the body's ability to process and transform nutrients into forms required for use by the body. Also, the nerves may become inflamed or undergo damage due to too much pressure being placed on the nerve due to various conditions.

Disease Type Peripheral Neuropathy

The most common cause of peripheral neuropathy falls into this category and is caused by diabetes. People suffering from diabetes sustain damage to the walls of blood vessels that supply blood to the nerves.

This impairs the normal blood flow and is a reason why many diabetics experience swelling in the calves, ankles and feet.

Over time, the altered blood flow starves the nerves of oxygen, eventually leading to peripheral neuropathy.

Other less common causes of peripheral neuropathy that fall into this category are autoimmune disorders like rheumatoid arthritis, inflammation of blood vessels (vasculitis), vitamin

B deficiency, viral or bacterial infections, and cancer.

Exposure Type Peripheral Neuropathy

In this type of peripheral neuropathy, your nerves have been exposed to toxins (poisonous substances created in living cells), or toxicants (artificial toxic substances) that damage the nerves.

One of the more common causes of peripheral neuropathy that falls into this category is a result of medication use. There is a surprising number of medications that are known to cause peripheral neuropathy.

Drugs that produce peripheral neuropathy include all of the following:

- Some cardiac drugs
- Statin drugs
- Blood pressure drugs
- Some cancer treatments (for example, chemotherapy)
- Psychiatric drugs
- Anti-seizure drugs
- Dermatitis treatment
- Anti-hypertensive drugs

- Cholesterol drugs

- Alcoholism treatment drugs

One Danish study reports that those on statin drugs are a staggering 14% more likely to develop peripheral neuropathy than those not on that type of medication.

Notice that this is quite a list that covers a wide range of medical conditions and may give us some insight as to why peripheral neuropathy is such a prevalent condition.

Another cause that falls into the exposure type of peripheral neuropathy is heavy alcohol consumption. Long term alcohol use in alcoholics creates a toxic environment for the nerves, leading to nerve damage. Damage to the liver also causes these individuals to become deficient in B vitamins, further complicating and adding to the severity of the condition.

Exposure to industrial toxic materials like mercury, lead, or arsenic may also create adverse conditions that lead to damage of the peripheral nerves, thereby causing neuropathy. There are many chemicals in wide use that have unknown health effects. It is possible that we will discover that there is a long list of chemicals that cause, among other things, neuropathy.

Traumatic Type Peripheral Neuropathy

As the name implies, direct trauma to the peripheral nerves can also cause peripheral neuropathy. The trauma can be either from a sudden injury like a car accident, or long term repetitive stress injuries, like those that develop "tennis elbow" from irritation of the nerves around the elbow. Some other examples of types of traumatic events that may cause this type of neuropathy are broken bones, sports injuries, major falls, spinal stenosis, or damage during surgery.

Chapter 4: Different Types of Peripheral Neuropathy

Peripheral neuropathy is generally associated with damage of the nerves specifically in the peripheral nervous system. This refers to damage to the nerves that are outside of the spinal cord and the brain. However, the central nervous system is not affected.

As discussed, peripheral neuropathy is caused by metabolic disorders like diabetes, exposure to toxins including certain medications, physical trauma, repetitive stress, infections, alcohol consumption, and many others.

Regardless of the cause of your peripheral neuropathy, not all nerves are affected in the same way. This is because in each nerve bundle there are actually several different types of nerves, each with different functions.

For example the nerves that regulate your heart activity aren't the same type of nerves that experience pain. The nerves that experience pain, aren't the same type of nerves that cause muscle contraction, allowing you to walk.

If all of these functions were done by one nerve, it would be more likely for signals to get crossed, causing confusion in the transmission of information between your body and your brain.

The three main types of nerves affected are motor nerves, sensory nerves and autonomic nerves. Because there are many different types of nerves, and many different causes of peripheral neuropathy, these nerves are affected to varying degrees in each person. In some, only one type of nerve is affected, others show signs that 2 types of nerves are affected, and still others exhibit evidence that all 3 types of nerves are affected.

I'm often asked why the nerves in the hands and feet are the most commonly affected, and the answer is fairly simple. These are the longest nerves, meaning they are the furthest from the spinal cord, which is not affected in peripheral neuropathy, and they are furthest from the heart, making them the most susceptible to swelling and changes in blood flow.

Read on to learn about the different types of nerves affected. And since it is so prevalent, I have also included a section specifically on diabetic peripheral neuropathy.

Sensory Nerve Neuropathy

One type of peripheral neuropathy affects your sensory nerves. Sensory nerves carry sensory information from the body back to the brain. As you can imagine, your body is being bombarded with sensory input all the time, and all of these senses "feel" a little different. This is because there are many different types of nerve receptors that respond differently depending on what is causing them to be stimulated.

We can break these types of receptors into 5 main categories which I will outline in detail. Knowing how your body responds to stimuli, and how a breakdown in the way that the nerve processes information due to nerve damage from peripheral neuropathy will make the next chapter on "Symptoms of Peripheral Neuropathy" make a lot more sense.

1. Mechanoreceptors

These types of receptors respond to mechanical forces. Some examples of mechanical forces are pressure, and vibration.

2. Thermoreceptors

These receptors are sensitive to changes in temperature

3. Chemoreceptors

These receptors are sensitive to chemical actions. Some examples are your taste buds and sense of smell.

4. Nociceptors

These are the pain sensors of the body. They are responsible for telling your brain when something is potentially damaging your body.

There are pain sensors for each of the above types of receptors. For example, there are pain sensors that respond to too much pressure (mechanoreceptors), to too much hot or cold (thermoreceptors), and chemical changes from tissue damage (chemoreceptors).

5. Photoreceptors

These respond to light and transmit the signal to the brain that we experience as vision.

In those with Sensory Nerve Peripheral Neuropathy, there can be changes to the way your brain receives and processes information from any of the senses listed above. With nerve damage that occurs with peripheral neuropathy these senses may become dulled, producing numbness, or they may become overly sensitive, causing the experience of pain from even the lightest touch.

Motor Nerve Peripheral Neuropathy

Motor nerves are the nerves that control muscles. This means that they control all voluntary movement of the body.

In those that have Motor Nerve Peripheral Neuropathy, their ability to move effectively has become affected. This can be due to muscle atrophy (shrinking of the muscles), muscle weakness, and reduced reflexes making walking and balance more difficult.

Autonomic Nerve Peripheral Neuropathy

Your autonomic nerves control the automatic functions in your body, meaning the functions not under your conscious control. This includes control of your internal organs and functions like heart rate, blood pressure, breathing and sweating.

With Autonomic Nerve Peripheral Neuropathy, it's scary to think, but these essential organs are affected.

This can lead to some pretty serious side effects, like heart arrhythmias or incontinence.

Even simple actions like swallowing food can become difficult.

More commonly, those with this type of peripheral neuropathy experience dizziness, gastrointestinal symptoms, and an inability to tolerate heat.

Diabetic Peripheral Neuropathy

I wanted to spend some extra time specifically addressing Diabetic Peripheral Neuropathy because it is the most common cause of peripheral neuropathy in the US.

This condition involves damage of the peripheral nerves in diabetic patients. The damage usually occurs as a result of high blood sugar over a long period of time (months to years). This eventually compromises many aspects of your health, so it is no surprise that the peripheral nerves are also affected.

Changes in blood flow cause damage to the cell walls of the nerves that supply much needed oxygen and nutrients to the peripheral nerves. Swelling in the feet can compress the nerves, further complicating the condition.

The symptoms come on slowly, and most people see it initially as just a minor annoyance. Over time, the symptoms progressively worsen. At that point there is wide variation in how each individual experiences their symptoms. It can range anywhere from a mild numbness, to a severe pain, or tingling and burning and everything in between.

Diabetic neuropathy usually affects the nerve fibers in the feet and legs. However, the condition could also be found affecting other parts of the body and presents with symptoms such as pain, numbness, dizziness, weakness, problems with balance, vision, the urinary tract system, digestive system, heart and the blood vessels.

From this, it's clear that Diabetic Peripheral Neuropathy can affect the Sensory Nervous System, Motor Nervous System and Autonomic Nervous System!

Diabetic neuropathy can be prevented by doing what it takes to keep your blood sugar under control and by living a healthy lifestyle.

Unfortunately many diabetic patients continue to experience neuropathy symptoms even after getting their blood sugar levels under control through medication. This is because the nerve damage has already taken place and additional steps need to be taken to stimulate the nerves and activate their healing cycle.

The good news is that by using proper treatment interventions, like the ones provided in my office, you can slow, stop and even reverse the progression of peripheral neuropathy. But time is the most important factor. The condition worsens every day you go without treatment, even if your symptoms remain the same for long periods of time.

If you have or suspect you have peripheral neuropathy, DO NOT WAIT to get checked out. My office info can be found at the end of this book.

Chapter 5: Peripheral Neuropathy Symptoms

People suffering from peripheral neuropathy can experience anything from one or two symptoms affecting just one type of nerve, to a large number of different symptoms affecting several different nerve pathways.

No two cases are exactly the same. This is because there are over 100 different known causes of peripheral neuropathy, and many different types of nerves that can be affected to varying degrees.

Sometimes the symptoms are hard to put into words because they are sensations that most people never experience making it difficult to categorize.

Often our patients will have to get creative when attempting to verbalize the true nature of their symptoms. They will use descriptions like, "It feels as if I have a glove or stocking on all the time", or, "It's like ants are crawling all over my feet", or even, "Every step is like I'm stepping on a bed of nails". Some experience pain only when they have shoes on, while others experience pain only when they have shoes off!

For this chapter I'm going to break the symptoms up into two sections. In the first, I will go over the more common or "classic" symptoms of peripheral neuropathy. In the second, I will provide a more comprehensive list of symptoms as they relate to each type of sensory, motor, or autonomic nerve. Finally, you can find a checklist at the end of the chapter where you can see how your symptoms correlate to the different types of nerves.

Classic Symptoms

The classic symptoms of peripheral neuropathy are those most commonly found in diabetics. This is simply due to the fact that diabetes is the most common cause of peripheral neuropathy in the United States.

Most experts agree that at least 50% of diabetics will experience peripheral neuropathy to a significant degree. Some groups even report numbers as high as 70%. This isn't to say that peripheral neuropathy sufferers who don't have diabetes won't have these exact same symptoms.

In fact, quite the opposite is true. Regardless of what the cause of the peripheral neuropathy is, whether it be diabetes, injury, medication toxicity, or idiopathic (no known cause), the typical or classic symptoms are the same. These are listed below:

- Numbness in the hands, legs or feet
- Sharp pain in the legs or feet
- Burning pain in the legs or feet
- Tingling or prickling in the legs or feet
- Extreme sensitivity to touch
- Reduced ability to tell the difference between hot and/or cold
- Muscle Cramps in the legs or feet
- Weakness in the legs or feet
- Pain with walking
- Pain and symptoms worse at night
- Dry or cracked skin on the feet
- Swelling in the legs, ankles or feet
- Inability to feel where you are stepping when you walk.

This is by no means a comprehensive list, but if you have even just one of these symptoms, it could be a sign that you have peripheral neuropathy and should get checked out as soon as possible. For a more comprehensive list, read below.

Comprehensive Symptom List

Your nerves control every function in your body so damage to your peripheral nerves can wreak havoc on your senses. What many don't realize is that in addition to your sensory nerves, your motor nerves that go to your muscles (and are usually under voluntary control), and your autonomic nerves that go to your internal organs (and are under involuntary control) can be equally affected. Listed here is a comprehensive list of potential symptoms as they relate to each of these nerve types.

Sensory Symptoms

- Sharp pains

- Numbness

- Tingling

- Burning

- Severe sensitivity to light touch

- Reduced ability to tell hot from cold

- Reduced or loss of reflexes
- Balance and coordination issues (due to inability to feel where your feet are in relation to your body)

Motor Symptoms

- Muscle weakness
- Muscle atrophy (shrinking of the muscles)
- Muscle cramps
- Involuntary muscle twitching
- Reduced or absent reflexes
- In severe cases, complete paralysis

Autonomic Symptoms

- Heat intolerance
- Noticeable changes in skin, nail, or hair
- Problems with swallowing
- Digestive Problems
  - Constipation
  - Diarrhea
- Dizziness
- Changes in blood pressure (orthostatic hypotension)

- Loss of ability to sweat

- Abnormal heart effects such as the heart beating too fast (Tachycardia)

- Urinary problems

- Sexual dysfunction

Persons exhibiting any of these symptoms should immediately consult a doctor for a full check-up. Treatment is dependent on many factors, but one thing is certain. The longer you wait to have treatment, the more your condition will progress, which will ultimately affect the expected outcomes.

Chapter 6: Major Complications of Peripheral Neuropathy

In earlier stages of peripheral neuropathy patients symptoms can range from annoying to unbearable. Regardless of where you fall on the scale, without proper treatment, peripheral neuropathy is a chronic progressive condition. This means that it's rare for it to self-correct and typically it will continue to worsen over time. As it worsens, there are some serious complications that may arise as a result.

For All Peripheral Neuropathy Sufferers

One of the most common major complications for those afflicted with peripheral neuropathy is an increased risk of falling. As the feet become numb, making it difficult to feel where your foot is hitting the ground, and you develop muscle weakness, affecting balance and coordination, your risk of falling steadily rises.

I want you to ask yourself: Have you ever known someone who has taken a major fall? For most, the answer is a resounding yes! How did it affect their life?

The statistics are staggering:

Falls are the #1 cause of death from injury in those over 65 years old

They account for about 9,500 deaths per year in the U.S.

25% of those who fall after the age of 65 and fracture a hip will die within 6 months

As you can see from this, treating peripheral neuropathy is about more than just trying to reduce symptoms. It can literally save your life.

For Diabetic Neuropathy Sufferers

In those 50-70% of diabetics that suffer from peripheral neuropathy, a major complication is diabetic ulcers or other injuries to the foot. As diabetic neuropathy progresses, you lose sensation to the feet. Because of this, the normal signals from your foot telling you that something is wrong never reach your brain.

Ulcers, cuts or blisters from shoes go completely unnoticed making them more prone to infection, and poor circulation makes them unlikely to heal on their own. Infection leads to further tissue damage and eventually gangrene.

In severe cases, amputation of the limb is the only option.

The Statistics

60% of adult non-traumatic lower limb amputations occur in those diagnosed with diabetes

This accounts for over 70,000 amputations per year.

The goal of a proper peripheral neuropathy treatment protocol is to regain the sensation in your feet. This will increase your body's ability to communicate these critical signals with your brain. With proper nerve signaling you can reduce the incidence of ulcers going unnoticed and ultimately reduce your risk of amputation.

Chapter 7: Treatment Options Part 1: The Traditional Medical Approach

In this chapter I will discuss some treatment options for peripheral neuropathy but I first want to distinguish between the different categories of treatment and goals of each category.

The first category of treatment is the traditional medical approach. The goal of these treatments is to manage symptoms. While some treatments are excellent at managing symptoms, giving much needed relief from pain, unfortunately they do nothing to heal the nerves that have been damaged.

The second category of treatment that will be discussed in the next chapter (Chapter 8: Treatment Options Part 2: The Conservative Approach, Nerve Regeneration and Neuropathy Reversal) is the conservative, or non-medical approach. It is called this because no medications or surgical interventions are used as part of the treatment. The ultimate goal of treatments in this category is to create the ideal conditions to help your nerves regenerate, thereby reversing your peripheral neuropathy.

These are the types of treatments utilized in my clinic and should always be considered if you have neuropathy symptoms.

Most with peripheral neuropathy have tried one or more medical interventions with varying degrees of success, so we will start by discussing them below.

The Traditional Medical Approach

Medical approaches to peripheral neuropathy can be divided into 2 categories: surgical and non-surgical methods.

Non-Surgical Methods: Medication

Non-surgical methods primarily involve prescription medication whose goal is to help relieve pain and other symptoms associated with peripheral neuropathy.

Below are listed some of the more common medications prescribed and what class of drug they fall into:

- Anti-seizure drugs
    - Gabapentin (Neurontin, Gralise)
    - Pregabalin (Lyrica)
- Anti-depressants
    - Amitryptaline
    - Doxepin
    - Nortriptyline (Pamelor)
    - Duloxetine (Cymbalta)
- Pain Relievers
    - Oxycontin
- Anti-inflammatories
    - Ibuprofin
    - Tylenol

These medications can help to alleviate symptoms and for some offer short term pain management. Sadly, for others the medication has no effect on reducing their pain, or reduces it for a short period but loses its effectiveness over time. This is because these medications don't treat the underlying cause of neuropathy symptoms, so the condition progresses over time.

Non-surgical methods: Injections

Another non-surgical medical approach is to administer nerve block injections. These nerve blocks act by interrupting transmission of the pain signal from the limbs to the brain. While there are no long term benefits to nerve block injections for neuropathy, they can provide short term pain relief.

Both medications and injections can do wonders in helping to alleviate neuropathy symptoms for short spans of time.

The challenge that I have found is that these medications can make it difficult to properly evaluate the full extent that the neuropathy has progressed. Covering up these symptoms may mask the true nature of the disease making it possible for the condition to be continually worsening, but without your knowledge.

Surgical Methods

Surgical methods consist of surgical decompression of compressed nerves in the affected areas. Surgical decompression has shown to have long term effects (based on 1 year follow up), but there are always potential risks and complications to surgery. Surgical intervention is only recommended in those that fail to respond to more conservative approaches.

Addressing Underlying Conditions

Regardless of whether you are receiving traditional medical treatments, or conservative non-medical treatment for your neuropathy, the best first step is to address any known underlying conditions.

A good example of this is in those who have peripheral neuropathy secondary to diabetes. Getting the diabetes under control should be considered either before or in conjunction with treatments for the neuropathy. This will both improve your overall health as well as help to make the neuropathy treatments more effective.

Some readers might be saying to themselves, "But my diabetes has been under control for years!", or "My chemotherapy has already ended", so "Why haven't my neuropathy symptoms improved on their own?"

There is a simple explanation for this:

While the original cause of the peripheral neuropathy (high blood sugar levels due to diabetes, or toxins from chemotherapy) is under control, this only prevents the neuropathy from progressing further. It does nothing to actually heal the nerves that have already been damaged.

At this point, the damage to the nerves has already been done. Treatments aimed at creating the ideal environment for nerve growth and regeneration are necessary to improve your symptoms and reverse this condition.

Treatments aimed at achieving this goal are outlined in the next chapter.

Chapter 8: Treatment Options Part 2: Conservative Approaches, Nerve Regrowth and Neuropathy Reversal

"Peripheral nerves have the ability to regenerate axons, as long as the nerve cell itself has not died, which may lead to functional recovery over time"

-National Institute of Neurologic Disorders and Stroke on the topic of Peripheral Neuropathy

I start this chapter by restating the quote from the introduction of this book because I think it's a powerful message of hope to those who think there are no options in treating or reversing their peripheral neuropathy. They have been told that their only option is medication to help alleviate their symptoms, and that their nerves have died or are dying and that there is no way for them to heal.

The National Institute of Neurologic Disorders and Stroke is a branch of the National Institute of Health and is a leading authority on research involving nerve conditions like peripheral neuropathy. Their message is clear that **nerves can regenerate** and **function can be restored**. We just need to create the ideal environment for the nerves to thrive.

I have always looked at treating peripheral neuropathy as being more than just trying to help with a collection of symptoms. What I am really trying to do is improve my patient's quality of life. For some, the pain and numbness is unbearable and they come to me at the end of their rope. Nothing else they have tried has been effective, and not only are their symptoms not getting any better, but they are getting steadily worse. They are at a greater risk of developing ulcers and gangrene which can lead to limb amputation, and they are at greater risk of falling, which can lead to death.

The reality is that not all peripheral neuropathy patients can be helped. Some have progressed so far that no amount of treatment will reverse their neuropathy and for those that can be helped, we may never reach 100% return to function. But for these sufferers, even 50% improvement can significantly improve their quality of life. Allowing them to have relief from pain, walk easier and sleep better while at the same time reducing the chance of amputation due to ulceration, or death due to falling.

Not everyone is a good candidate for these treatments, but for those who are, the results can be truly life changing. While there is no universal cure for peripheral neuropathy, one thing is clear: Without proper treatment **the condition will worsen.**

As stated in the previous chapter, the goal of this approach to neuropathy treatment is two-fold: Improve symptoms like pain, numbness, tingling and burning, while at the same time regenerating damaged nerves and reversing the neuropathy.

If you are already on medication to help manage your neuropathy symptoms, it's important that you consult with your prescribing physician before reducing your dosage, or stopping altogether.

In my clinic we work closely with our patient's medical providers to ensure that we develop and deliver the most safe and effective peripheral neuropathy treatments consistent with the most up to date research and treatment modalities.

When I talk about conservative or non-medical approaches to neuropathy treatment, I'm referring to methods that don't require the use of drugs or surgery. The goal of these therapies is to treat the underlying causes of the neuropathy in order to achieve lasting benefits.

Listed below are the types of treatments I use in my office that I have found to be the most effective at providing long term improvement in neuropathy symptoms.

I don't want to give the reader any impression that the conservative approach is easy. In fact, it takes a commitment from both the patient and the provider to see a care plan through to completion.

Unlike medicine and injections which can offer immediate relief, with conservative care each treatment session builds on the previous treatment and the effects are cumulative over time. The reason why we use this approach in my office is we can see **true functional improvement** which ultimately leads to **long lasting relief**.

While no two treatments are exactly the same, I have found that by taking a multidirectional approach we can see the greatest gains.

Laser Therapy

One of the most recent breakthroughs in the treatment of neuropathy is the use of a specially designed therapeutic laser.

This type of therapy treatment, nicknamed Low Level Laser Therapy, or "Cold Laser" therapy, I've found to be especially effective in treatment of neuropathy. This type of laser is specifically designed to be non-ablative (non-surgical) because the laser light travels through the skin without doing any damage to the tissue or causing any excess heat.

The highest power lasers for therapeutic use are Class IV lasers and are FDA approved for treatment of pain. These Class IV lasers, though non-ablative, are still very powerful and are strictly regulated for use by qualified health professionals.

The special laser light stimulates the deep tissue and works by improving circulation and activating 3 cellular mechanisms. The first mechanism reduces inflammation in the tissues and the area around the nerve. The second mechanism calms the nerve by naturally bringing the Sodium and Potassium levels back into balance (controls nerve firing). The last and most important mechanism actually stimulates your body's own natural healing process. It provides much needed

ATP, which is the energy source for all cellular processes, aiding in nerve regeneration.

Infrared Light Therapy

Light therapy using infrared LEDs has been effective as a general treatment across the spectrum of different types of neuropathy.

An LED light "boot" or blanket is used on the affected areas. Infrared therapy stimulates the release of nitric oxide. This dilates the blood vessels which increases circulation. The sudden increase in circulation brings much needed nutrients to the nerves, assisting in their healing process. It has been shown to reduce both pain and numbness in neuropathy sufferers.

Mechanical Vibration

There is evidence showing that applying low-level mechanical vibration to the skin, at specific frequencies, can significantly enhance tactile sensitivity (ability to sense touch).

Stimulation is applied to the foot, with care being taken to establish and observe a sensitivity threshold.

The mechanisms behind improvement aren't fully understood, but this kind of vibration may add mechanical energy to enhance your body's ability to transmit sensation through the dermal tissue.

It may also change the so-called "pain gate" in the spinal cord to help with nerve function, further restoring tactile sensitivity.

The treatment involves standing on a specialized vibrating platform, which activates the body's stretch reflex for spontaneous muscle contraction. This spontaneous muscle contraction pumps much needed blood to the affected areas, stimulates nerve impulses and helps to restore both muscle strength and coordination.

Electrical Nerve Stimulation

In this form of treatment, electrodes are attached to the skin while a gentle yet powerful current is delivered to the affected areas at varying frequencies.

There are many different types of electrical muscle stimulation therapies. What I have found to be most effective is a specific type of muscle stimulation device that causes involuntary contraction of the muscles in the treated areas. This muscle contraction is rarely achieved (and can be dangerous) in home devices and should only be done under the direction of a trained healthcare provider. The action of this type of electrical stimulation is to pump blood down into the hands or feet and simultaneously stimulate the affected nerves.

Compression Massage Therapy

For many with peripheral neuropathy, massage therapy has been shown to be one of the most effective ways to manage and reduce pain. Massage can be done manually or with assisted devices and acts by helping to improve circulation, reduce swelling, increase range of motion and reduce pressure on the nerves.

Physical Therapy

Physical Therapy can help in releasing nerve entrapment, improve strength, balance, coordination and flexibility.

Topical Creams

The advantage of these kinds of creams is that they can be applied directly to the pain site, where they act as local anesthetics, numbing the site to provide relief.

Many of these products contain capsaicin, a painkiller derived from chili peppers, while others use botanical oils.

There is also a medical grade topical cream available from my office which relies on a menthol base and is very effective at relieving symptoms.

Neuropathy Support Supplements

This is a broad category that includes vitamin supplementation as well as holistic and dietary approaches to manage neuropathy symptoms and aid in nerve regrowth.

The nutritional approach should only be implemented under the supervision of a qualified healthcare professional.

Nutritional approaches are most effective when combined with specific dietary modifications and in conjunction with other treatments listed in this chapter.

Not all vitamins are created equal and there is mounting evidence showing that vitamins and herbs sold over the counter at major retail outlets lack the quality control to accurately label their products. In essence, what you are paying for may not be what you are actually getting. The highest quality vitamins and nutritional supplements with strict quality control standards are only offered through healthcare professionals.

There are literally hundreds of nutritional supplements available, but the most effective formula I have found combines alpha lipoic acid, benfotiamine and methylcobalamine into a single pharmaceutical grade, natural supportive product. Research shows that benfotiamine and methylcoboalamine can assist in reducing symptoms, while alpha lipoic acid can improve nerve conduction.

Other promising possibilities include B12 shots (which can actually cure neuropathy if it is caused by a severe B12 deficiency), acetyl-L-carnitine, and gamma linolenic acid.

Curcumin, geranium oil, evening primrose oil, and fish oil supplements with omega-3 fatty acids may also help alleviate symptoms.

See the next chapter for more detailed info on natural options for symptom reduction.

Chapter 9: Natural Options for Reducing Neuropathy Symptoms

According to a report released by the Neuropathy Association, an estimated 20 million individuals suffer from mild to severe forms of peripheral neuropathy.

This painful and debilitating condition can significantly decrease a patient's quality of life and can result in serious complications.

As listed in Chapter 7, there are a great many medications that are used to control the symptoms of neuropathy. But there are also numerous natural supplements that have been proven to reduce the symptoms without the side effects associated with many medications.

Here are some of the natural options:

Benfotiamine

This is a man-made form of vitamin B1 (thiamine), a vitamin that is essential for nerves to function properly.

Taking a vitamin B1 supplement ensures that the body has adequate levels of B1, which can result in a decrease in the symptoms of neuropathy.

It has been shown to be particularly effective in decreasing pain associated with diabetic neuropathy and it also reduces microvascular damage that results from frequent high blood sugar levels.

Vitamin B2

Vitamin B2 (riboflavin) is an antioxidant that works to make certain the nervous system is properly functioning and fights off free radicals in the body that cause pain.

Physicians have found that having a deficient amount of vitamin B2 can lead to or worsen the symptoms of peripheral neuropathy.

This vitamin is easily obtained in supplement form. There are also many foods that are rich in B2, like leafy greens, broccoli, cauliflower, Brussels sprouts, peppers, and squash.

Try adding them to your diet.

Vitamin B6

Vitamin B6 (pyridoxine), is an essential vitamin that is required in sufficient levels for fat, carbohydrate, and protein metabolism.

Deficient levels in the body can result in fatigue, moodiness, irritability, and neuropathy.

Researchers have found that almost all diabetics suffering from neuropathy have a vitamin B6 deficiency resulting in worsening symptoms.

Supplementation to bring vitamin B6 back to normal levels may help reduce neuropathy symptoms. It can also be found in foods like sunflower seeds, pistachios and tuna fish.

Vitamin B12

Vitamin B12 (methylcobalamine) is necessary to protect the body against neurological diseases.

High levels of methylcobalamine have been proven to regenerate neurons and the myelin sheath that provides protection for the nerve axons and peripheral nerves.

Patients that have received injections of vitamin B12 in the form of methylcobalamine have reported decreased neuropathy symptoms as well as improved balance and less weakness.

Also try foods like seafood, beef and eggs.

Vitamin D

Vitamin D promotes nerve and neuron growth. Deficient levels of Vitamin D have been determined to impair pain receptor function, increase the potential for nerve damage, and to be a risk factor for diabetic neuropathy.

Recent research has found that Vitamin D supplementation can slow down progression of peripheral neuropathy and significantly decreases the amount of neuropathic pain felt.

Vitamin D is usually accompanied by vitamin A because they act synergistically to suppress cells that produce inflammatory chemicals. Vitamin D and A are also used together to combat other disorders like autoimmune disease.

Sun exposure has long been known to help the body produce its own vitamin D.

R-Alpha Lipoic Acid

R-Alpha Lipoic Acid is an antioxidant produced by the body and found in all cells.

Studies have shown that its effectiveness at killing free radicals proves beneficial to patients suffering from peripheral neuropathy.

Patients report decreased burning, tingling, itching, and numbness associated with nerve damage.

Natural Herbs

There are also numerous herbs available that have the potential to be beneficial in the reduction of neuropathy symptoms.

Feverfew Extract has been found to help control the symptoms of neuropathy, specifically nerve pain.

Oat Straw Extract acts to decrease general pain, nerve pain, and helps sooth the itchy skin that some patients develop with Neuropathy.

Skullcap Extract works to cause a tranquilizing effect on the nervous system. It has a tremendous impact on decreasing neuropathy symptoms including pain and tingling.

Finally, Flower Passion is an herb that has been found to eliminate symptoms especially nerve pain. Many patients take more than one supplement for maximum relief.

Before beginning any supplements it is essential to speak with your physician to find out if there may be any possible interactions with your current medicine regimen and to determine what dosages are appropriate for you.

Be aware that most patients report that it takes approximately three weeks to begin seeing the benefits associated with taking these supplements, and the most dramatic improvements involve proper supplementation in conjunction with dietary modifications and other conservative treatments.

Chapter 10: Peripheral Neuropathy and Lifestyle

Changes You Can Make Today To Reduce Neuropathy Symptoms

Living with neuropathy pain every day is not only uncomfortable, but affects mood as well. It is not uncommon for chronic neuropathy sufferers to experience depression.

The medical industry has identified over 100 known types of nerve pain. In America today, about 3% of the population suffers from some form of nerve pain and its symptoms. Symptoms include numbness or tingling in the extremities, the degree of which can range from moderate to severe.

The sufferer may experience painful "pins and needles" sensations in the feet or hands and fingers. Feelings of intense heat or cold due to decreased circulation in the limbs are other possible symptoms. Ongoing nerve pain is the basis for diagnosing patients with neuropathy.

This pain and other symptoms of neuropathy can affect one's ability to go about functioning normally in their everyday life.

However, making a few simple lifestyle changes can limit the risk of one's health from spiraling downward into further decline.

One common side effect of peripheral neuropathy is for the sufferer to become less active due to pain. The less active the person is, the greater the chance that chronic pain will restrict mobility.

The last thing a patient typically wants is to become bed ridden, so the faster you can make lifestyle changes to reduce neuropathy symptoms, the better chances you have for maintaining a happy and productive life.

Change Your Diet

People living with neuropathy and its symptoms should begin by changing their diet.

One of the most important dietary changes to make is to include more fruits and vegetables. In fact, one should switch over to a diet heavy in vegetables.

Eat lots of green leafy vegetables and be sure to add more of the darker fruits such as blueberries, pomegranates, purple grapes and black plumbs to the diet. This ensures the body gets enough of the vitamins, minerals and antioxidants it needs to support health and energy levels.

Stop Smoking

Smoking constricts blood vessels that supply nutrients to the nerves, thereby increasing neuropathy symptoms. Smoking cessation can help to reduce neuropathy symptoms.

Stop the Consumption of Alcohol

Alcohol use can cause damage to peripheral nerves and may lead to vitamin deficiencies that further worsen neuropathy symptoms. Stopping or reducing alcohol consumption can both reduce symptoms associated with neuropathy, as well as prevent the condition from progressing further.

Add an Exercise Routine

Exercising is very important. It helps keep the body limber and the muscles strong. Before beginning, take the time to learn how to exercise properly to avoid injury and do not forget to do a warm up before exercising and a cool down afterward.

Get at least two 15 minute sessions of moderate exercise in each day. Low impact exercises are best, such as walking and swimming.

Wear Loose Clothing and Shoes

Tight socks and shoes can cause poor circulation in the feet and legs. Wear loose-fitting clothes to help reduce pain and symptoms.

Wear the proper footwear that your doctor recommends for people who have neuropathy pain in the feet.

Eating right, exercising the right way, and wearing the right type of clothing, are important lifestyle changes to make to reduce neuropathy pain and other symptoms.

10 Quick Facts (In Case You Missed Them)

1. There are over 100 different causes of Peripheral Neuropathy.

2. It is estimated to affect 4%-6% of those over 55 years of age.

3. The most common symptoms are pain, tingling, numbness, burning and/or weakness in the feet or hands.

4. The #1 cause in the U.S. is Diabetes.

5. An estimated 50%-70% of diabetics suffer from peripheral neuropathy.

6. Complications of peripheral neuropathy can lead to limb amputation, falls, paralysis and death.

7. Traditional Medical Approaches provide symptomatic relief while the condition worsens.

8. There are natural options to reduce neuropathy symptoms without drugs or surgery.

9. Conservative Approaches (outlined in this book) stimulate nerve growth and regeneration.

10. Reversing Peripheral Neuropathy IS Possible!

Conclusion

Peripheral Neuropathy is a chronic condition of the nerves affecting 20 million people in the U.S. alone. There are over 100 known causes of neuropathy, with metabolic conditions such as diabetes and nerve damage from prescription medication or chemotherapy being the most prevalent. Half of all diabetics will experience symptoms associated with peripheral neuropathy. An estimated 30% of peripheral neuropathy cases are considered "idiopathic", meaning there is no known cause.

Regardless of the cause, peripheral neuropathy can be a debilitating condition that significantly hinders the sufferer's quality of life. With symptoms such as pain, burning, numbness, tingling, weakness, and balance issues, it's no wonder sufferers are desperate to find a solution.

Those with peripheral neuropathy are more likely to have to undergo limb amputations, and they have a significantly increased risk of falling, which can ultimately lead to death in those over 65 years of age.

Most readers of this are already taking some form of medication for their peripheral neuropathy. Common medications include Gabapentin (**Neurontin, Gralise**), Pregabalin (**Lyrica**) and Duloxetine (**Cymbalta**).

While these medications may help ease the symptoms of peripheral neuropathy, they do nothing to treat the cause of the neuropathy which allows the condition to worsen over time.

Neuropathy can be reversed!

Targeted treatments, like those offered in our office, focus on restoring proper blood flow, supplying vital nutrients and stimulated your body's own natural healing process. Utilizing cutting edge technology like FDA approved Laser Therapy, Infrared therapy, compression massage, electrical nerve stimulation, vibration therapy and medical grade vitamin therapy, your nerves can heal and actually regrow parts that have started to die off.

Because peripheral neuropathy is a chronic progressive condition, one thing is clear: **Without proper treatment, the condition will worsen**. If you have peripheral neuropathy, DON'T WAIT TO GET TREATMENT! Nerves that have completely died off cannot be regenerated, so whether you've had neuropathy for 10 weeks or 10 years, the sooner you start treatment the better your chances of success.

To Schedule a Peripheral Neuropathy Consultation:

Call 301-907-6533 and mention this book to schedule a free neuropathy consultation in our Bethesda, Maryland office.

Welcome To The
Easy-To Read Section

The following is a reprint of the book, *Reversing Peripheral Neuropathy*.

This book is two books in one, or rather, it is one book printed twice.

The first (approx.) half is the book printed with normal lay-out conventions which makes it the easiest way for many people to read the book.

Peripheral Neuropathy, as you will learn, afflicts a wide range of people.

A good many have their best eyesight behind them. To address this we have changed the lay-out and have adopted larger print and formatting rules that are the latest in easy to read type.

The book has then been reprinted and reformatted with large easy to read type and with font selection, spacing and other formatting specifically designed to allow the reader, who would normally have trouble reading "normal" printed text, to read comfortably and easily.

Table of Contents

Introduction

"Peripheral nerves have the ability to regenerate axons, as long as the nerve cell itself has not died, which may lead to functional recovery over time"

-National Institute of Neurologic Disorders and Stroke on the topic of Peripheral Neuropathy

I start the introduction to this book with the above quote because nearly every patient who comes into my office has heard from at least one doctor (and usually multiple doctors) that:

1) There is nothing that can be done for Peripheral Neuropathy other than medication to manage symptoms.

2) Their condition will only get worse.

3) Nerves can't regenerate.

They come for their initial examination with a skeptical mind but out of desperation to find some relief (ANY relief) from the pain, numbness, tingling and/or burning in their feet. For most, nothing else they have tried has seemed to be able to help.

So I start with this quote to inspire hope! One of the most prominent authorities on neurologic disorders, a division of the National Institute of Health is saying, "Yes, peripheral nerves can regenerate", and "Yes, nerves damaged due to peripheral neuropathy can return to normal function".

It's an exciting job I have to be able to restore hope to those who feel hopeless. To deliver treatment options to those who thought there were none.

In this book, *Reversing Peripheral Neuropathy*, you will learn about the many causes of peripheral neuropathy, why traditional approaches to treatment have failed, and what can be done to take back control of your condition and your life.

Chapter 1: What is Peripheral Neuropathy?

Peripheral Neuropathy is a condition in which a person experiences pain, numbness, tingling, burning and/or weakness, usually in the hands and feet, though it may occur in other parts of the body.

The word itself betrays the general and somewhat mysterious nature of the disease. "Neuro-", meaning related to nerves and "-pathy", pertaining to a disease or ailment. In medical circles, one can see that a lot of different conditions could be attributed to "something wrong with the nerves."

Regardless of the vague definition, peripheral neuropathy (also sometimes referred to as polyneuropathy) is typically diagnosed when a person has pain or numbness where there is no direct or observable cause for it.

This can occur as a result of nerve damage in the peripheral nervous system, which essentially encompasses all parts of the nervous system outside of the brain and spinal cord (i.e. spinal nerves).

These nerves are responsible for communicating information from the body back through the spinal cord and eventually to the brain.

As the nerves become more and more damaged, the normal signals become muted (numbness, weakness), or altered (pain, tingling, burning). These types of "nerve symptoms" are signs that the nerves are beginning to die.

There are 3 main types of nerves that can be affected to varying degrees:

Autonomic nerves: These regulate heart rate, sweating, blood pressure and other automatic functions of the body.

Motor nerves: These control the body muscles and are usually under conscious control.

Sensory nerves: These transmit sensations (such as pain, touch, heat and cold) from other body parts to the brain.

Some peripheral neuropathy sufferers will exhibit symptoms related to only one of these nerve types, while others will have symptoms related to two nerve types, and still others will show signs and symptoms of damage to all 3 nerve types.

Read on to find more on some of the common causes of this condition.

Chapter 2: Diagnosing Peripheral Neuropathy

There are over 100 causes and dozens of symptoms that can be associated with peripheral neuropathy, so it is important that the clinician be familiar with all of them in order to make the appropriate clinical correlation.

Many diabetic patients or those in the early stages of peripheral neuropathy are often asymptomatic. However, properly trained healthcare professionals can still identify slight tell-tale signs of the condition.

Specialized clinical tests can help determine what the general health condition of the patient is.

It may reveal the underlying cause of your peripheral neuropathy which will aid the doctor in developing an appropriate treatment plan and what the expected outcomes will be after treatment.

Physicians look out for the following Diabetic Neuropathy symptoms:

- Reduced ankle reflexes
- Painless foot injuries
- Infections
- Gangrene

The diagnosing of peripheral neuropathy usually starts with a symptoms survey. This will give the clinician a detailed account of what you are experiencing and how it has changed or progressed over time.

The next step in diagnosing peripheral neuropathy is to perform a detailed neurological exam. Although this exam is comprehensive, it is fairly straightforward and does not necessarily require expensive equipment or scans.

In my office we use tried and true methods of determining to what degree you can still feel the affected limbs. We test your ability to feel vibration, temperature, tactile and other sensory perceptions.

These methods are all simple yet very effective in determining which nerves have been affected by your peripheral neuropathy and to what degree. Many of our patients are shocked to see first-hand how far along their peripheral neuropathy has progressed!

Using a standard scoring system we can then calculate how much function you have lost in your peripheral nerves. This gives us an objective measure to easily track your progress throughout the treatment.

We then use a highly specialized foot scanner to take a 3-D image of your foot. This gives us an up close view to evaluate for ulcers or other changes to the structure of the feet.

It measures pressure from side to side so we can evaluate specific pressure points, which may be relieved with specialized orthotic devices. Lastly, it measures the heat signature across the foot. An area of increased heat is a tell-tale sign of increased inflammation which helps us to determine a starting point for delivering treatment.

Other Diagnostic Methods

In Neurology offices, sometimes electrodiagnostic tools are used to assess peripheral neuropathies.

The first is called an Electromyogram, or EMG for short. This test measures the electrical activity of the muscles.

The second is called Nerve Conduction Velocity Study, or NCV for short. This test measures how fast a nerve can send an electric signal.

These two tests together are useful in determining the overall health of the muscles and nerves. They can show which nerves are affected by peripheral neuropathy and to what extent they have been affected.

By using electrodiagnostics, the doctor can determine an expected prognosis for the patient. As long as there is still some nerve function, it tells us that the nerve is not completely dead, meaning that the prognosis for recovery is good. If there is no nerve function, meaning that the lesion is definitive, recovery will be limited.

In either case, early intervention is key in maximizing results with treatment.

Chapter 3: What Causes Peripheral Neuropathy?

Peripheral neuropathy is fairly common in people over the age of 55. Approximately 4% to 6% of the people in this age group showed signs and symptoms of the disorder. Those with metabolic syndromes like diabetes are at a significantly greater risk with estimates that over 50% of diabetics suffer from peripheral neuropathy to some degree.

Over 100 different types of peripheral neuropathy have been

identified and it is caused by many different underlying conditions.

In most cases, the disease damages nerves in the peripheral nervous system, usually in the hands and feet, but spares the brain and spinal cord.

Causes of peripheral neuropathy can be divided into 3 main categories: Disease type, Exposure type and Traumatic type, which we will discuss in this chapter.

It is important to note that although these 3 categories exist, many cases of peripheral neuropathy are considered "idiopathic", meaning that there is no known cause.

The symptoms and effects of idiopathic peripheral neuropathy are the same as those found in other neuropathy sufferers, and treatments are equally effective across the groups.

Regardless of which category your peripheral neuropathy falls into, one of the root causes is damage to the small blood vessels that supply the nerves.

This starves the nerve of essential oxygen and nutrients which in turn results in nerve damage and the eventual dying off of the nerve.

Think of it as if the peripheral nerves in your hands or feet were like the roots of a tree and your blood supply is the tree's water source. What would happen if you stopped watering the roots of a tree?

It would start to die! And that is exactly what happens to your nerves when they are starved of their blood supply. The symptoms associated with peripheral neuropathy are a result of this withering of the nerves. This is an important point to remember for later in the book when I discuss different treatment options.

Besides being starved of oxygen, systemic diseases may affect the body's ability to process and transform nutrients into forms required for use by the body. Also, the nerves may become inflamed or undergo damage due to too much pressure being placed on the nerve due to various conditions.

Disease Type Peripheral Neuropathy

The most common cause of peripheral neuropathy falls into this category and is caused by diabetes. People suffering from diabetes sustain damage to the walls of blood vessels that supply blood to the nerves.

This impairs the normal blood flow and is a reason why many diabetics experience swelling in the calves, ankles and feet.

Over time, the altered blood flow starves the nerves of oxygen, eventually leading to peripheral neuropathy.

Other less common causes of peripheral neuropathy that fall into this category are autoimmune disorders like rheumatoid arthritis, inflammation of blood vessels (vasculitis), vitamin B deficiency, viral or bacterial infections, and cancer.

Exposure Type Peripheral Neuropathy

In this type of peripheral neuropathy, your nerves have been exposed to toxins (poisonous substances created in living cells), or toxicants (artificial toxic substances) that damage the nerves.

One of the more common causes of peripheral neuropathy that falls into this category is a result of medication use. There is a surprising number of medications that are known to cause peripheral neuropathy.

Drugs that produce peripheral neuropathy include all of the following:

- Some cardiac drugs
- Statin drugs
- Blood pressure drugs
- Some cancer treatments (for example, chemotherapy)
- Psychiatric drugs
- Anti-seizure drugs
- Dermatitis treatment

- Anti-hypertensive drugs

- Cholesterol drugs

- Alcoholism treatment drugs

One Danish study reports that those on statin drugs are a staggering 14% more likely to develop peripheral neuropathy than those not on that type of medication.

Notice that this is quite a list that covers a wide range of medical conditions and may give us some insight as to why peripheral neuropathy is such a prevalent condition.

Another cause that falls into the exposure type of peripheral neuropathy is heavy alcohol consumption. Long term alcohol use in alcoholics creates a toxic environment for the nerves, leading to nerve damage. Damage to the liver also causes these individuals to become deficient in B vitamins, further complicating and adding to the severity of the condition.

Exposure to industrial toxic materials like mercury, lead, or arsenic may also create adverse conditions that lead to damage of the peripheral nerves, thereby causing neuropathy.

Traumatic Type Peripheral Neuropathy

As the name implies, direct trauma to the peripheral nerves can also cause peripheral neuropathy. The trauma can be either from a sudden injury like a car accident, or long term repetitive stress injuries, like those that develop "tennis elbow" from irritation of the nerves around the elbow. Some other examples of types of traumatic events that may cause this type of neuropathy are broken bones, sports injuries, major falls, spinal stenosis, or damage during surgery.

Chapter 4: Different Types of Peripheral Neuropathy

Peripheral neuropathy is generally associated with damage of the nerves specifically in the peripheral nervous system. This refers to damage to the nerves that are outside of the spinal cord and the brain. However, the central nervous system is not affected.

As discussed, peripheral neuropathy is caused by metabolic disorders like diabetes, exposure to toxins including certain medications, physical trauma, repetitive stress, infections, alcohol consumption, and many others.

Regardless of the cause of your peripheral neuropathy, not all nerves are affected in the same way. This is because in each nerve bundle there are actually several different types of nerves, each with different functions.

For example the nerves that regulate your heart activity aren't the same type of nerves that experience pain. The nerves that experience pain, aren't the same type of nerves that cause muscle contraction, allowing you to walk.

If all of these functions were done by one nerve, it would be more likely for signals to get crossed, causing confusion in the transmission of information between your body and your brain.

The three main types of nerves affected are motor nerves, sensory nerves and autonomic nerves. Because there are many different types of nerves, and many different causes of peripheral neuropathy, these nerves are affected to varying degrees in each person. In some, only one type of nerve is affected, others show signs that 2 types of nerves are affected, and still others exhibit evidence that all 3 types of nerves are affected.

I'm often asked why the nerves in the hands and feet are the most commonly affected, and the answer is fairly simple. These are the longest nerves, meaning they are the furthest from the spinal cord, which is not affected in peripheral neuropathy, and they are furthest from the heart, making them the most susceptible to swelling and changes in blood flow.

Read on to learn about the different types of nerves affected. And since it is so prevalent, I have also included a section specifically on diabetic peripheral neuropathy.

Sensory Nerve Neuropathy

One type of peripheral neuropathy affects your sensory nerves. Sensory nerves carry sensory information from the body back to the brain. As you can imagine, your body is being bombarded with sensory input all the time, and all of these senses "feel" a little different. This is because there are many different types of nerve receptors that respond differently depending on what is causing them to be stimulated.

We can break these types of receptors into 5 main categories which I will outline in detail.

Knowing how your body responds to stimuli, and how a breakdown in the way that the nerve processes information due to nerve damage from peripheral neuropathy will make the next chapter on "Symptoms of Peripheral Neuropathy" make a lot more sense.

1) Mechanoreceptors

These types of receptors respond to mechanical forces. Some examples of mechanical forces are pressure, and vibration.

2) Thermoreceptors

These receptors are sensitive to changes in temperature. Damage to these is common.

3) Chemoreceptors

These receptors are sensitive to chemical actions. Some examples are your taste buds and sense of smell.

4) Nociceptors

These are the pain sensors of the body. They are responsible for telling your brain when something is potentially damaging your body.

There are pain sensors for each of the above types of receptors. For example, there are pain sensors that respond to too much pressure (mechanoreceptors), to too much hot or cold (thermoreceptors), and chemical changes from tissue damage (chemoreceptors).

5) Photoreceptors

These respond to light and transmit the signal to the brain that we experience as vision.

In those with Sensory Nerve Peripheral Neuropathy, there can be changes to the way your brain receives and processes information from any of the senses listed above.

With nerve damage that occurs with peripheral neuropathy these senses may become dulled, producing numbness, or they may become overly sensitive, causing the experience of pain from even the lightest touch.

Motor Nerve Peripheral Neuropathy

Motor nerves are the nerves that control muscles. This means that they control all voluntary movement of the body.

In those that have Motor Nerve Peripheral Neuropathy, their ability to move effectively has become affected. This can be due to muscle atrophy (shrinking of the muscles), muscle weakness, and reduced reflexes making walking and balance more difficult.

Autonomic Nerve Peripheral Neuropathy

Your autonomic nerves control the automatic functions in your body, meaning the functions not under your conscious control. This includes control of your internal organs and functions like heart rate, blood pressure, breathing and sweating.

With Autonomic Nerve Peripheral Neuropathy, it's scary to think, but these essential organs are affected.

This can lead to some pretty serious side effects, like heart arrhythmias or incontinence. Even simple actions like swallowing food can become difficult.

More commonly, those with this type of peripheral neuropathy experience dizziness, an inability to tolerate heat and gastrointestinal symptoms.

Diabetic Peripheral Neuropathy

I wanted to spend some extra time specifically addressing Diabetic Peripheral Neuropathy because it is the most common cause of peripheral neuropathy in the US.

This condition involves damage of the peripheral nerves in diabetic patients. The damage usually occurs as a result of high blood sugar over a long period of time (months to years). This eventually compromises many aspects of your health, so it is no surprise that the peripheral nerves are also affected.

Changes in blood flow cause damage to the cell walls of the nerves that supply much needed oxygen and nutrients to the peripheral nerves.

Swelling in the feet can compress the nerves, further complicating the condition.

The symptoms come on slowly, and most people see it initially as just a minor annoyance. Over time, the symptoms progressively worsen. At that point there is wide variation in how each individual experiences their symptoms. It can range anywhere from a mild numbness, to a severe pain, or tingling and burning and everything in between.

Diabetic neuropathy usually affects the nerve fibers in the feet and legs. However, the condition could also be found affecting other parts of the body and presents with symptoms such as pain, numbness, dizziness, weakness, problems with balance, vision, the urinary tract system, digestive system, heart and the blood vessels.

From this, it's clear that Diabetic Peripheral Neuropathy can affect the Sensory Nervous System, Motor Nervous System and Autonomic Nervous System!

Diabetic neuropathy can be prevented by doing what it takes to keep your blood sugar under control and by living a healthy lifestyle.

Unfortunately many diabetic patients continue to experience neuropathy symptoms even after getting their blood sugar levels under control through medication. This is because the nerve damage has already taken place and additional steps need to be taken to stimulate the nerves and activate their healing cycle.

The good news is that by using proper treatment interventions, like the ones provided in my office, you can slow, stop and even reverse the progression of peripheral neuropathy. But time is the most important factor. The condition worsens every day you go without treatment, even if your symptoms remain the same for long periods of time.

If you have or suspect you have peripheral neuropathy, DO NOT WAIT to get checked out. My office info can be found at the end of this book.

Chapter 5: Peripheral Neuropathy Symptoms

People suffering from peripheral neuropathy can experience anything from one or two symptoms affecting just one type of nerve, to a large number of different symptoms affecting several different nerve pathways.

No two cases are exactly the same. This is because there are over 100 different known causes of peripheral neuropathy, and many different types of nerves that can be affected to varying degrees.

Sometimes the symptoms are hard to put into words because they are sensations that most people never experience making it difficult to categorize.

Often our patients will have to get creative when attempting to verbalize the true nature of their symptoms. They will use descriptions like, "It feels as if I have a glove or stocking on all the time", or, "It's like ants are crawling all over my feet", or even, "Every step is like I'm stepping on a bed of nails". Some experience pain only when they have shoes on, while others experience pain only when they have shoes off!

For this chapter I'm going to break the symptoms up into two sections. In the first, I will go over the more common or "classic" symptoms of peripheral neuropathy.

In the second, I will provide a more comprehensive list of symptoms as they relate to each type of sensory, motor, or autonomic nerve. Finally, you can find a checklist at the end of the chapter where you can see how your symptoms correlate to the different types of nerves.

Classic Symptoms

The classic symptoms of peripheral neuropathy are those most commonly found in diabetics. This is simply due to the fact that diabetes is the most common cause of peripheral neuropathy in the United States.

Most experts agree that at least 50% of diabetics will experience peripheral neuropathy to a significant degree. Some groups even report numbers as high as 70%. This isn't to say that peripheral neuropathy sufferers who don't have diabetes won't have these exact same symptoms.

In fact, quite the opposite is true. Regardless of what the cause of the peripheral neuropathy is, whether it be diabetes, injury, medication toxicity, or idiopathic (no known cause), the typical or classic symptoms are the same. These are listed below:

- Numbness in the hands, legs or feet

- Sharp pain in the legs or feet

- Burning pain in the legs or feet

- Tingling or prickling in the legs or feet

- Extreme sensitivity to touch

- Reduced ability to tell the difference between hot and/or cold

- Muscle Cramps in the legs or feet

- Weakness in the legs or feet

- Pain with walking

- Pain and symptoms worse at night

- Dry or cracked skin on the feet

- Swelling in the legs, ankles or feet

- Inability to feel where you are stepping when you walk.

This is by no means a comprehensive list, but if you have even just one of these symptoms, it could be a sign that you have peripheral neuropathy and should get checked out as soon as possible.

For a more comprehensive list, read below.

Comprehensive Symptom List

Your nerves control every function in your body so damage to your peripheral nerves can wreak havoc on your senses. What many don't realize is that in addition to your sensory nerves, your motor nerves that go to your muscles (and are usually under voluntary control), and your autonomic nerves that go to your internal organs (and are under involuntary control) can be equally affected. Listed here is a comprehensive list of potential symptoms as they relate to each of these nerve types.

Sensory Symptoms

- Sharp pains
- Numbness

- Tingling
- Burning
- Severe sensitivity to light touch
- Reduced ability to tell hot from cold
- Reduced or loss of reflexes
- Balance and coordination issues (due to inability to feel where your feet are in relation to your body)

Motor Symptoms

- Muscle weakness
- Muscle atrophy (shrinking of the muscles)
- Muscle cramps
- Involuntary muscle twitching
- Reduced or absent reflexes

- In severe cases, complete paralysis

Autonomic Symptoms

- Heat intolerance
- Noticeable changes in skin, nail, or hair
- Problems with swallowing
- Digestive Problems
  - Constipation
  - Diarrhea
- Dizziness
- Changes in blood pressure (orthostatic hypotension)
- Loss of ability to sweat
- Abnormal heart effects such as the heart beating too fast (Tachycardia)
- Urinary problems

- Sexual dysfunction

Persons exhibiting any of these symptoms should immediately consult a doctor for a full check-up. Treatment is dependent on many factors, but one thing is certain. The longer you wait to have treatment, the more your condition will progress, which will ultimately affect the expected outcomes.

Chapter 6: Major Complications of Peripheral Neuropathy

In earlier stages of peripheral neuropathy patients symptoms can range from annoying to unbearable. Regardless of where you fall on the scale, without proper treatment, peripheral neuropathy is a chronic progressive condition. This means that it's rare for it to self-correct and typically it will continue to worsen over time. As it worsens, there are some serious complications that may arise as a result.

For All Peripheral Neuropathy Sufferers

One of the most common major complications for those afflicted with peripheral neuropathy is an increased risk of falling. As the feet become numb, making it difficult to feel where your foot is hitting the ground, and you develop muscle weakness, affecting balance and coordination, your risk of falling steadily rises.

I want you to ask yourself: Have you ever known someone who has taken a major fall? For most, the answer is a resounding yes! How did it affect their life?

The statistics are staggering:

Falls are the #1 cause of death from injury in those over 65 years old

They account for about 9,500 deaths per year in the U.S.

25% of those who fall after the age of 65 and fracture a hip will die within 6 months

As you can see from this, treating peripheral neuropathy is about more than just trying to reduce symptoms. It can literally save your life.

For Diabetic Neuropathy Sufferers

In those 50-70% of diabetics that suffer from peripheral neuropathy, a major complication is diabetic ulcers or other injuries to the foot. As diabetic neuropathy progresses, you lose sensation to the feet. Because of this, the normal signals from your foot telling you that something is wrong never reach your brain.

Ulcers, cuts or blisters from shoes go completely unnoticed making them more prone to infection, and poor circulation makes them unlikely to heal on their own. Infection leads to further tissue damage and eventually gangrene.

In severe cases, amputation of the limb is the only option.

60% of adult non-traumatic lower limb amputations occur in those diagnosed with diabetes

This accounts for over 70,000 amputations per year.

The goal of a proper peripheral neuropathy treatment protocol is to regain the sensation in your feet. This will increase your body's ability to communicate these critical signals with your brain. With proper nerve signaling you can reduce the incidence of ulcers going unnoticed and ultimately reduce your risk of amputation.

Chapter 7:
Treatment Options Part 1:
The Traditional Medical Approach

In this chapter I will discuss some treatment options for peripheral neuropathy but I first want to distinguish between the different categories of treatment and goals of each category.

The first category of treatment is the traditional medical approach. The goal of these treatments is to manage symptoms. While some treatments are excellent at managing symptoms, giving much needed relief from pain, unfortunately they do nothing to heal the nerves that have been damaged.

The second category of treatment that will be discussed in the next chapter (Chapter 8: Treatment Options Part 2: The Conservative Approach, Nerve Regeneration and Neuropathy Reversal) is the conservative, or non-medical approach. It is called this because no medications or surgical interventions are used as part of the treatment. The ultimate goal of treatments in this category is to create the ideal conditions to help your nerves regenerate, thereby reversing your peripheral neuropathy.

These are the types of treatments utilized in my clinic and should always be considered if you have neuropathy symptoms.

Most with peripheral neuropathy have tried one or more medical interventions with varying degrees of success, so we will start by discussing them below.

The Traditional Medical Approach

Medical approaches to peripheral neuropathy can be divided into 2 categories: surgical and non-surgical methods.

Non-Surgical Methods: Medication

Non-surgical methods primarily involve prescription medication whose goal is to help relieve pain and other symptoms associated with peripheral neuropathy.

Below are listed some of the more common medications prescribed and what class of drug they fall into:

- Anti-seizure drugs
    - Gabapentin (Neurontin, Gralise)
    - Pregabalin (Lyrica)
- Anti-depressants
    - Amitryptaline
    - Doxepin
    - Nortriptyline (Pamelor)
    - Duloxetine (Cymbalta)
- Pain Relievers
    - Oxycontin
- Anti-inflammatories
    - Ibuprofin
    - Tylenol

These medications can help to alleviate symptoms and for some offer short term pain management. Sadly, for others the medication has no effect on reducing their pain, or reduces it for a short period but loses its effectiveness over time. This is because these medications don't treat the underlying cause of neuropathy symptoms, so the condition progresses over time.

Non-surgical methods: Injections

Another non-surgical medical approach is to administer nerve block injections. These nerve blocks act by interrupting transmission of the pain signal from the limbs to the brain. While there are no long term benefits to nerve block injections for neuropathy, they can provide short term pain relief.

Both medications and injections can do wonders in helping to alleviate neuropathy symptoms for short spans of time.

The challenge that I have found is that these medications can make it difficult to properly evaluate the full extent that the neuropathy has progressed. Covering up these symptoms may mask the true nature of the disease making it possible for the condition to be continually worsening, but without your knowledge.

Surgical Methods

Surgical methods consist of surgical decompression of compressed nerves in the affected areas. Surgical decompression has shown to have long term effects (based on 1 year follow up), but there are always potential risks and complications to surgery. Surgical intervention is only recommended in those that fail to respond to more conservative approaches.

Addressing Underlying Conditions

Regardless of whether you are receiving traditional medical treatments, or conservative non-medical treatment for your neuropathy, the best first step is to address any known underlying conditions.

A good example of this is in those who have peripheral neuropathy secondary to diabetes. Getting the diabetes under control should be considered either before or in conjunction with treatments for the neuropathy. This will both improve your overall health as well as help to make the neuropathy treatments more effective.

Some readers might be saying to themselves, "But my diabetes has been under control for years!", or "My chemotherapy has already ended", so "Why haven't my neuropathy symptoms improved on their own?"

There is a simple explanation for this:

While the original cause of the peripheral neuropathy (high blood sugar levels due to diabetes, or toxins from chemotherapy) is under control, this only prevents the neuropathy from progressing further. It does nothing to actually heal the nerves that have already been damaged.

At this point, the damage to the nerves has already been done. Treatments aimed at creating the ideal environment for nerve growth and regeneration are necessary to improve your symptoms and reverse this condition.

Treatments aimed at achieving this goal are outlined in the next chapter.

Chapter 8:
Treatment Options Part 2: Conservative Approaches, Nerve Regrowth and Neuropathy Reversal

"Peripheral nerves have the ability to regenerate axons, as long as the nerve cell itself has not died, which may lead to functional recovery over time"

-National Institute of Neurologic Disorders and Stroke on the topic of Peripheral Neuropathy

I start this chapter by restating the quote from the introduction of this book because I think it's a powerful message of hope to those who think there are no options in treating or reversing their peripheral neuropathy. They have been told that their only option is medication to help alleviate their symptoms, and that their nerves have died or are dying and that there is no way for them to heal.

The National Institute of Neurologic Disorders and Stroke is a branch of the National Institute of Health and is a leading authority on research involving nerve conditions like peripheral neuropathy. Their message is clear that nerves can regenerate and function can be restored. We just need to create the ideal environment for the nerves to thrive.

I have always looked at treating peripheral neuropathy as being more than just trying to help with a collection of symptoms. What I am really trying to do is improve my patient's quality of life. For some, the pain and numbness is unbearable and they come to me at the end of their rope. Nothing else they have tried has been effective, and not only are their symptoms not getting any better, but they are getting steadily worse. They are at a greater risk of developing ulcers and gangrene which can lead to limb amputation, and they are at greater risk of falling, which can lead to death.

The reality is that not all peripheral neuropathy patients can be helped. Some have progressed so far that no amount of treatment will reverse their neuropathy and for those that can be helped, we may never reach 100% return to function. But for these sufferers, even 50% improvement can significantly improve their quality of life. Allowing them to have relief from pain, walk easier and sleep better while at the same time reducing the chance of amputation due to ulceration, or death due to falling.

Not everyone is a good candidate for these treatments, but for those who are, the results can be truly life changing. While there is no universal cure for peripheral neuropathy, one thing is clear: Without proper treatment the condition will worsen.

As stated in the previous chapter, the goal of this approach to neuropathy treatment is two-fold: Improve symptoms like pain, numbness, tingling and burning, while at the same time regenerating damaged nerves and reversing the neuropathy.

If you are already on medication to help manage your neuropathy symptoms, it's important that you consult with your prescribing physician before reducing your dosage, or stopping altogether.

In my clinic we work closely with our patient's medical providers to ensure that we develop and deliver the most safe and effective peripheral neuropathy treatments consistent with the most up to date research and treatment modalities.

When I talk about conservative or non-medical approaches to neuropathy treatment, I'm referring to methods that don't require the use of drugs or surgery. The goal of these therapies is to treat the underlying causes of the neuropathy in order to achieve lasting benefits.

Listed below are the types of treatments I use in my office that I have found to be the most effective at providing long term improvement in neuropathy symptoms.

I don't want to give the reader any impression that the conservative approach is easy. In fact, it takes a commitment from both the patient and the provider to see a care plan through to completion.

Unlike medicine and injections which can offer immediate relief, with conservative care each treatment session builds on the previous treatment and the effects are cumulative over time. The reason why we use this approach in my office is we can see true functional improvement which ultimately leads to long lasting relief.

While no two treatments are exactly the same, I have found that by taking a multidirectional approach we can see the greatest gains.

Laser Therapy

One of the most recent breakthroughs in the treatment of neuropathy is the use of a specially designed therapeutic laser.

This type of therapy treatment, nicknamed Low Level Laser Therapy, or "Cold Laser" therapy, I've found to be especially effective in treatment of neuropathy. This type of laser is specifically designed to be non-ablative (non-surgical) because the laser light travels through the skin without doing any damage to the tissue or causing any excess heat.

The highest power lasers for therapeutic use are Class IV lasers and are FDA approved for treatment of pain. These Class IV lasers, though non-ablative, are still very powerful and are strictly regulated for use by qualified health professionals.

The special laser light stimulates the deep tissue and works by improving circulation and activating 3 cellular mechanisms. The first mechanism reduces inflammation in the tissues and the area around the nerve. The second mechanism calms the nerve by naturally bringing the Sodium and Potassium levels back into balance (controls nerve firing). The last and most important mechanism actually stimulates your body's own natural healing process. It provides much needed ATP, which is the energy source for all cellular processes, aiding in nerve regeneration.

Infrared Light Therapy

Light therapy using infrared LEDs has been effective as a general treatment across the spectrum of different types of neuropathy.

An LED light "boot" or blanket is used on the affected areas. Infrared therapy stimulates the release of nitric oxide. This dilates the blood vessels which increases circulation.

The sudden increase in circulation brings much needed nutrients to the nerves, assisting in their healing process.

This type of therapy has been shown to reduce both pain and numbness in neuropathy sufferers and is growing in popularity among doctors who treat neuropathy.

Mechanical Vibration

There is evidence showing that applying low-level mechanical vibration to the skin, at specific frequencies, can significantly enhance tactile sensitivity (ability to sense touch).

Stimulation is applied to the foot, with care being taken to establish and observe a sensitivity threshold.

The mechanisms behind improvement aren't fully understood, but this kind of vibration may add mechanical energy to enhance your body's ability to transmit sensation through the dermal tissue.

It may also change the so-called "pain gate" in the spinal cord to help with nerve function, further restoring tactile sensitivity.

The treatment involves standing on a specialized vibrating platform, which activates the body's stretch reflex for spontaneous muscle contraction. This spontaneous muscle contraction pumps much needed blood to the affected areas, stimulates nerve impulses and helps to restore both muscle strength and coordination.

Electrical Nerve Stimulation

In this form of treatment, electrodes are attached to the skin while a gentle yet powerful current is delivered to the affected areas at varying frequencies.

There are many different types of electrical muscle stimulation therapies. What I have found to be most effective is a specific type of muscle stimulation device that causes involuntary contraction of the muscles in the treated areas. This muscle contraction is rarely achieved (and can be dangerous) in home devices and should only be done under the direction of a trained healthcare provider. The action of this type of electrical stimulation is to pump blood down into the hands or feet and simultaneously stimulate the affected nerves.

Compression Massage Therapy

For many with peripheral neuropathy, massage therapy has been shown to be one of the most effective ways to manage and reduce pain.

Massage can be done manually or with assisted devices and acts by helping to improve circulation, reduce swelling, increase range of motion and reduce pressure on the nerves.

Physical Therapy

Physical Therapy can help in releasing nerve entrapment, improve strength, balance, coordination and flexibility.

Topical Creams

The advantage of these kinds of creams is that they can be applied directly to the pain site, where they act as local anesthetics, numbing the site to provide relief.

Many of these products contain capsaicin, a painkiller derived from chili peppers, while others use botanical oils.

There is also a medical grade topical cream available from my office which relies on a menthol base and is very effective at relieving the painful symptoms of peripheral neuropathy.

Neuropathy Support Supplements

This is a broad category that includes vitamin supplementation as well as holistic and dietary approaches to manage neuropathy symptoms and aid in nerve regrowth.

The nutritional approach should only be implemented under the supervision of a qualified healthcare professional.

Nutritional approaches are most effective when combined with specific dietary modifications and in conjunction with other treatments listed in this chapter.

Not all vitamins are created equal and there is mounting evidence showing that vitamins and herbs sold over the counter at major retail outlets lack the quality control to accurately label their products. In essence, what you are paying for may not be what you are actually getting. The highest quality vitamins and nutritional supplements with strict quality control standards are only offered through healthcare professionals.

There are literally hundreds of nutritional supplements available, but the most effective formula I have found combines alpha lipoic acid, benfotiamine and methylcobalamine into a single pharmaceutical grade, natural supportive product. Research shows that benfotiamine and methylcoboalamine can assist in reducing symptoms, while alpha lipoic acid can improve nerve conduction.

Other promising possibilities include B12 shots (which can actually cure neuropathy if it is caused by a severe B12 deficiency), acetyl-L-carnitine, and gamma linolenic acid.

Curcumin, geranium oil, evening primrose oil, and fish oil supplements with omega-3 fatty acids may also help alleviate symptoms.

See the next chapter for more detailed info on natural options for symptom reduction.

Chapter 9: Natural Options for Reducing Neuropathy Symptoms

According to a report released by the Neuropathy Association, an estimated 20 million individuals suffer from mild to severe forms of peripheral neuropathy.

This painful and debilitating condition can significantly decrease a patient's quality of life and can result in serious complications.

As listed in Chapter 7, there are a great many medications that are used to control the symptoms of neuropathy. But there are also numerous natural supplements that have been proven to reduce the symptoms without the side effects associated with many medications.

Here are some of the natural options:

Benfotiamine

This is a man-made form of vitamin B1 (thiamine), a vitamin that is essential for nerves to function properly.

Taking a vitamin B1 supplement ensures that the body has adequate levels of B1, which can result in a decrease in the symptoms of neuropathy.

It has been shown to be particularly effective in decreasing pain associated with diabetic neuropathy and it also reduces microvascular damage that results from frequent high blood sugar levels.

Vitamin B2

Vitamin B2 (riboflavin) is an antioxidant that works to make certain the nervous system is properly functioning and fights off free radicals in the body that cause pain.

Physicians have found that having a deficient amount of vitamin B2 can lead to or worsen the symptoms of peripheral neuropathy.

This vitamin is easily obtained in supplement form. There are also many foods that are rich in B2, like leafy greens, broccoli, cauliflower, Brussels sprouts, peppers, and squash.

Try adding them to your diet.

Vitamin B6

Vitamin B6 (pyridoxine), is an essential vitamin that is required in sufficient levels for fat, carbohydrate, and protein metabolism.

Deficient levels in the body can result in fatigue, moodiness, irritability, cracks around the mouth, depression, confusion, anemia, and neuropathy.

Researchers have found that almost all diabetics suffering from neuropathy have a vitamin B6 deficiency resulting in worsening symptoms.

Supplementation to bring vitamin B6 back to normal levels may help reduce neuropathy symptoms. Vitamin B6 can also be found in foods like sunflower seeds, pistachios and tuna fish.

Vitamin B12

Vitamin B12 (methylcobalamine) is necessary to protect the body against neurological diseases.

High levels of methylcobalamine have been proven to regenerate neurons and the myelin sheath that provides protection for the nerve axons and peripheral nerves.

Patients that have received injections of vitamin B12 in the form of methylcobalamine have reported decreased neuropathy symptoms as well as improved balance and less weakness.

Also try foods like seafood, beef and eggs.

Vitamin D

Vitamin D promotes nerve and neuron growth. Deficient levels of Vitamin D have been determined to impair pain receptor function, increase the potential for nerve damage, and to be a risk factor for diabetic neuropathy.

Recent research has found that Vitamin D supplementation can slow down progression of peripheral neuropathy and significantly decreases the amount of neuropathic pain felt.

Vitamin D is usually accompanied by vitamin A because they act synergistically to suppress cells that produce inflammatory chemicals.

Vitamin D and A are also used together to combat other disorders like autoimmune disease.

Sun exposure has long been known to help the body produce its own vitamin D.

R-Alpha Lipoic Acid

R-Alpha Lipoic Acid is an antioxidant produced by the body and found in all cells.

Studies have shown that its effectiveness at killing free radicals proves beneficial to patients suffering from peripheral neuropathy.

Patients report decreased burning, tingling, itching, and numbness associated with nerve damage.

Natural Herbs

There are also numerous herbs available that have the potential to be beneficial in the reduction of neuropathy symptoms.

Feverfew Extract has been found to help control the symptoms of neuropathy, specifically nerve pain.

Oat Straw Extract acts to decrease general pain, nerve pain, and helps sooth the itchy skin that some patients develop with Neuropathy.

Skullcap Extract works to cause a tranquilizing effect on the nervous system. It has a tremendous impact on decreasing neuropathy symptoms including pain and tingling.

Finally, Flower Passion is an herb that has been found to eliminate symptoms especially nerve pain. Many patients take more than one supplement for maximum relief.

Before beginning any supplements it is essential to speak with your physician to find out if there may be any possible interactions with your current medicine regimen and to determine what dosages are appropriate for you.

Be aware that most patients report that it takes approximately three weeks to begin seeing the benefits associated with taking these supplements, and the most dramatic improvements involve proper supplementation in conjunction with dietary modifications and other conservative treatments.

Chapter 10: Peripheral Neuropathy and Lifestyle

Changes You Can Make Today To Reduce Neuropathy Symptoms

Living with neuropathy pain every day is not only uncomfortable, but affects mood as well. It is not uncommon for chronic neuropathy sufferers to experience depression.

The medical industry has identified over 100 known types of nerve pain. In America today, about 3% of the population suffers from some form of nerve pain and its symptoms. Symptoms include numbness or tingling in the extremities, the degree of which can range from moderate to severe.

The sufferer may experience painful "pins and needles" sensations in the feet or hands and fingers. Feelings of intense heat or cold due to decreased circulation in the limbs are other possible symptoms. Ongoing nerve pain is the basis for diagnosing patients with neuropathy.

This pain and other symptoms of neuropathy can affect one's ability to go about functioning normally in their everyday life.

However, making a few simple lifestyle changes can limit the risk of one's health from spiraling downward into further decline.

One common side effect of peripheral neuropathy is for the sufferer to become less active due to pain. The less active the person is, the greater the chance that chronic pain will restrict mobility.

The last thing a patient typically wants is to become bed ridden, so the faster you can make lifestyle changes to reduce neuropathy symptoms, the better chances you have for maintaining a happy and productive life.

Change Your Diet

People living with neuropathy and its symptoms should begin by changing their diet.

One of the most important dietary changes to make is to include more fruits and vegetables. In fact, one should switch over to a diet heavy in vegetables.

Eat lots of green leafy vegetables and be sure to add more of the darker fruits such as blueberries, pomegranates, purple grapes and black plumbs to the diet. This ensures the body gets enough of the vitamins, minerals and antioxidants it needs to support health and energy levels.

Stop Smoking

Smoking constricts blood vessels that supply nutrients to the nerves, thereby increasing neuropathy symptoms. Smoking cessation can help to reduce neuropathy symptoms.

Stop the Consumption of Alcohol

Alcohol use can cause damage to peripheral nerves and may lead to vitamin deficiencies that further worsen neuropathy symptoms.

Stopping or reducing alcohol consumption can both reduce symptoms associated with neuropathy, as well as prevent the condition from progressing further.

Add an Exercise Routine

Exercising is very important. It helps keep the body limber and the muscles strong.

Before beginning, take the time to learn how to exercise properly to avoid injury and do not forget to do a warm up before exercising and a cool down afterward. Part of your warm up should include stretching. Stretching will help prevent injuries, especially in the beginning.

Get at least two 15 minute sessions of moderate exercise in each day. Low impact exercises are best, such as walking and swimming.

Wear Loose Clothing and Shoes

Tight socks and shoes can cause poor circulation in the feet and legs. Wear loose-fitting clothes to help reduce pain and symptoms.

Wear the proper footwear that your doctor recommends for people who have neuropathy pain in the feet.

Eating right, exercising the right way, and wearing the right type of clothing, are important lifestyle changes to make to reduce neuropathy pain and other symptoms.

10 Quick Facts (In Case You Missed Them)

1. There are over 100 different causes of Peripheral Neuropathy.
2. It is estimated to affect 4%-6% of those over 55 years of age.
3. The most common symptoms are pain, tingling, numbness, burning and/or weakness in the feet or hands.
4. The #1 cause in the U.S. is Diabetes.

5. An estimated 50%-70% of diabetics suffer from peripheral neuropathy.

6. Complications of peripheral neuropathy can lead to limb amputation, falls, paralysis and death.

7. Traditional Medical Approaches provide symptomatic relief while the condition worsens.

8. There are natural options to reduce neuropathy symptoms without drugs or surgery.

9. Conservative Approaches (outlined in this book) stimulate nerve growth and regeneration.

10. Reversing Peripheral Neuropathy IS Possible

Conclusion

Peripheral Neuropathy is a chronic condition of the nerves affecting 20 million people in the U.S. alone. There are over 100 known causes of neuropathy, with metabolic conditions such as diabetes and nerve damage from prescription medication or chemotherapy being the most prevalent. Half of all diabetics will experience symptoms associated with peripheral neuropathy. An estimated 30% of peripheral neuropathy cases are considered "idiopathic", meaning there is no known cause.

Regardless of the cause, peripheral neuropathy can be a debilitating condition that significantly hinders the sufferer's quality of life. With symptoms such as pain, burning, numbness, tingling, weakness, and balance issues, it's no wonder sufferers are desperate to find a solution.

Those with peripheral neuropathy are more likely to have to undergo limb amputations, and they have a significantly increased risk of falling, which can ultimately lead to death in those over 65 years of age.

Most readers of this are already taking some form of medication for their peripheral neuropathy. Common medications include Gabapentin (**Neurontin, Gralise**), Pregabalin (**Lyrica**) and Duloxetine (**Cymbalta**).

While these medications may help ease the symptoms of peripheral neuropathy, they do nothing to treat the cause of the neuropathy which allows the condition to worsen over time.

Neuropathy can be reversed!

Targeted treatments, like those offered in our office, focus on restoring proper blood flow, supplying vital nutrients and stimulated your body's own natural healing process.

Utilizing cutting edge technology like FDA approved Laser Therapy, Infrared therapy, compression massage, electrical nerve stimulation, vibration therapy and medical grade vitamin therapy, your nerves can heal and actually regrow parts that have started to die off.

Because peripheral neuropathy is a chronic progressive condition, one thing is clear: **Without proper treatment, the condition will worsen**. If you have peripheral neuropathy, DON'T WAIT TO GET TREATMENT! Nerves that have completely died off cannot be regenerated, so whether you've had neuropathy for 10 weeks or 10 years, the sooner you start treatment the better your chances of success.

To Schedule Your Peripheral Neuropathy Consultation:

Call 301-907-6533 and mention this book to schedule a free neuropathy consultation in our Bethesda, Maryland office.

INDEX

Made in the USA
San Bernardino, CA
05 November 2016